A SELF-HELP GUIDE FOR UNDERSTANDING CANCER

DR BHRATRI BHUSHAN

MBBS, MD (INTERNAL MEDICINE),
DM (MEDICAL ONCOLOGY)
CONSULTANT MEDICAL ONCOLOGIST

FIRST EDITION

CONTENTS

*"One person caring about another repre-
sents life's greatest value."*
Jim Rohn

PREFACE

I should clarify that this book is not a textbook, nor is it a comprehensive guide for the uninitiated. It is a light hearted book and my sole purpose of writing this book is to do my part in war against cancer; using a tool that I like the most apart from practicing medical oncology, writing. This book is inspired not by cutting edge research and wonders of modern medical science but by the patients and their families sitting in front of me over the years.

Cancer is a powerful word and many people are more afraid of cancer than actually dying. This book then can serve to enhance understanding of the readers and to bring them up to speed to what means what in cancer, about the myths and misconceptions and about the things we can change. I want to dedicate this book to patients of cancer, as they have been my biggest teachers and their courage my inspiration. At the end of the day, it's all about healing and according to me, modern medicine should aspire to reduce human suffering above all else.

Special thanks to my father Dr Bharat Bhushan, mother Mrs Vimla, wife Dr Manju Bhushan, brother Bhuvan Bhushan, sister-in-law Namrata Vrishni, son Varchasv and niece Surkhi; without them nothing is possible in my life, let alone this book.

CHAPTER 1
INTRODUCTION

There are only a few other words in language that carry the same weight as the word *cancer*. It is a life altering experience to hear the words *"you have cancer"*. Also in the face of rising incidence of this deadly disease in every part of the world, we often fear of having this disease diagnosed in us or in our loved ones. It is one of the diseases that more often than not happens to be outside of our control. Money too is sometimes not the answer. The terminology, techniques and the sheer amount of the information patients and their relatives encounter is overwhelming; and in today's world often the onus of the responsibility of choosing among various options lies on patients.

Not long ago, I found myself on rounds during my undergraduate days, often encountering advanced stage cancer patients and I heard statements like *"nothing can be done"*, *"send him home on supportive and symptomatic medicines"* or *"explain and refer to some hospice setting"*, from my professors.

On the other end of the spectrum, there were cancer patients who were detected relatively early and they theoretically had excellent survival, with many of them having possibility of getting cured for life. They had an even bigger problem than the advanced stage of unfortunate patients, which was lack of knowledge and even general awareness. And despite counselling them extensively, they gave up hope just by knowing that they had cancer.

Then as I made progress in my career and did MD in internal medicine and then DM in medical oncology, newer therapies continued to evolve and more and more patients were offered therapies that were previously just not there. My knowledge grew, and patients became more aware, but even to this day I find the similar challenges of my undergrad days, although in different guise.

Cancer is not *one* disease. The science of cancer medicine is extremely complex, ever rapidly evolving. Decision making takes place after thorough interdisciplinary discussions and even the internationally accepted guidelines keep changing. So if I may give my reader my humble advice, it will be to have trust in modern medical science and your doctors. The best strategy is to get expert help as soon as possible and as long as needed, any deviation from this can lead to mismanagement. Cancers have a doubling time, a time in which cancer *becomes double* to whatever extent it is present today. This is different for different cancers, as a rule of thumb you can take three weeks as doubling time, so every three weeks delay in getting expert care will double the cancer and chances of cure will fall by just not half but exponentially.

What I like the most about modern medicine is that it is evidence based and it's very transparent. Honesty is the key in modern medical sciences, and there is no way around it. If a patient has a median overall survival of six months, then doctors have to inform the patient of the same and then discuss the potential benefits of various treatments. In the same way when the chances of cure are excellent, the same is conveyed. The basis of all the recommendations are randomised controlled clinical trials and/ or meta-analysis of trials, which are the highest possible scientific proof available. To top it all off, there are internationally accepted and followed guidelines that ought to be adhered to by treating physicians; any deviation from which has to be thoroughly explained and approved by a group of experts.

By *"trusting your doctor"*, I don't mean you should have blind faith.

Ask questions, as many as you can. Explore all the sources to educate yourself, consult as many specialists as you like. To educate the patient and to answer all the queries is one of the major responsibilities of the doctor. In fact the word doctor is derived from Latin *docere,* to teach. But you must never trust anyone who is not a qualified cancer specialist and be particularly aware of people who claim *"certain and guaranteed"* treatments, but can provide no evidence for their claims. Degrees matter for a reason. The word cancer means *crab*, and in the past it was envisioned as an ailment that starts at one point in body and slowly grabs the whole body by spreading to its various parts, like a crab would by it's limbs. To defeat this deadly disease the most important weapon is awareness. The expertise of the doctor coupled with the understanding of the general population, is the only way forward to any meaningful impact on human suffering due to cancer.

CHAPTER 2

CANCER ORIGINS, A DIFFERENT YOU

What makes cancer different from other diseases, is it's origins and basic nature. Most of the diseases are caused by something external, like bacteria, protozoans, fungus, virus etc. Many chronic diseases are caused by a failing system like heart, kidney, liver or brain. But cancer is unique, as no other disease arises from our own body having an *agenda, or a sort of a mind* of its own. Cancer is an organism that is part of the body, yet so different. It is like harboring a parasite which is the product of our own DNA, only with minor differences from normal cells.

This creates a unique situation and Darwin's evolutionary principles apply. It indeed becomes survival of the fittest and battle deciding the survivor is fought between the *normal you* and the *cancerous you.* This is the reason, why most of the cancer treatments are so toxic. The cells that we try to kill are our own cells, only with subtle differences in their biology.

Everybody develops millions of abnormal and potentially cancerous cells everyday, they just don't manifest as cancer because of our body's genetic defensive mechanisms and immune system. It has been postulated that everyday ten thousand mutations occur in us and they are contained and then corrected, if a mutation can't be corrected, then our immune system identifies and kills the defective cells. Cancer research is a fascinating field, how an abnormal cell develops and then survives to give rise to almost a new *entity* inside us, which then competes with our own bodies and develops mechanisms so strong that it ends up killing the host!

Darwin's natural selection works in these situations and in the battle between cancer and normal tissue, the fittest survives. Most of the times, as we already discussed cancer cells are destroyed and there are no consequences. But sometimes a unique set of abnormal cells arises and it gives rise to more cells, they form lumps and they grow in size until the cell volume reaches a critical mass and the cancer becomes clinically diagnosable. Cancers are detectable with conventional methods when they weigh about one gram, which is equivalent to one billion cancer cells. This is an oversimplification, but if a patient can be detected at the earliest stage possible they have at least one billion cancer cells and when these one gram of cancer cells divide, eventually becoming about one kilogram of cancer cells, that is one thousand billion cells, then it is fatal for the patient.

Cancer cells are abnormal, from their visual appearance to their genetic makeup. There are minor differences from normal cells, but these minor differences get in a sort of chain reaction and everything changes. Cancer is not just a simple growth, it is a smart growth. There are many types of *lumps* that are not cancerous, they just stay where they are and while they grow in size, they don't *invade* the normal tissues of the host. The problem with cancer is its propensity to spread; if cancers were just confined to where they started from then there wouldn't have been such a death toll associated with this disease.

Body tries to kill cancer cells and under the pressure of survival these abnormal cells develop ingenious ways to propagate themselves. More and more mutations take place. Once cancer cells reach a critical mass, it becomes difficult for them to sustain their nutritional needs, so they *hack* one of the most potent tools of human biology: *angiogenesis,* which means formation of new blood vessels. So, now the cancer tissue gets its own blood supply via these self-made blood vessels, which are attached to normal ones. The system is not as perfect and harmonious as normal vascular system, but for the time being it sustains cancer.

As the cell number grows, it becomes difficult for the cancer to survive on this newly formed, defective blood vessel network; so parts of it begin to die and once again under the pressure of survival, they develop the most devastating capability: to *metastasize,* to spread. They can spread by direct spread, lymphatic system or it can be via blood stream. Now the cancer cells perform a tremendous feat, they leave their tissue of origin (say, lung) and go to an entirely different organ (like liver or brain) and they start living there. So with time not only the organ of origin is slowly engulfed by cancer but other vital organs too. After sometime the vital functions of the body start to become compromised and the critical level is reached after which the patient dies.

The therapeutic modalities used in cancer patients are directed to these pathways of cancer progression. Surgery primarily aims to remove the disease in the organ of origin as well as in the metastatic sites, if possible. Radiation is more versatile and can reach sites where surgery tends to be difficult and morbid. Radiation is often used to cover the margins of a surgical field, to reduce chances of local recurrence and also to kill cancerous deposits at metastatic sites for the relief of pain and other symptoms, among its other uses. Chemotherapy is used after surgery (adjuvant) to eliminate the cells that have already reached at other sites, but are not manifest yet. It can be used to reduce the size of cancer to make it more amenable to be cured by other modalities (neoadjuvant). In widespread disease, chemo functions by eliminating as much cells as possible to extend the lifespan (palliative).

Chemotherapy and its functions depend on mathematical

models; if a chemo kills 99.9% of all cancer cells, still millions of cancer cells are left behind. If we combine two chemotherapies then the cell kill is enhanced but it can never reach to 100%, because there are many other factors in play, like the adaptability of cancer cells, ongoing mutations and resistance patterns. There have been explosive advancements in field of cancer medicine and especially in the recent years with more advanced molecules developed than ever. There is a term increasingly being used, *pathological complete response*, which means that after being given chemotherapy or chemoradiation, surgery was performed and the final analysis of the surgical specimen showed no tumor; so, there was a *complete response.* But still, chemo has its primary role as an adjunctive strategy in the curative setting; although by itself it is not the approach which can solely cure solid cancers. Although there are exceptions like choriocarcinoma. On the other hand chemo is the only curative approach for hematological (blood) malignancies like leukaemia, lymphoma and myeloma, in which it is highly successful.

CHAPTER 3
HABITS AND CANCER,
WHAT WE CAN DO

Longevity is great, in fact it is one of the most important indications of how well a society or a nation is doing, but it comes with an inevitable evil: cancer. Cancer, no matter what type is associated with aging and the more the age, more is the incidence of a particular type of cancer; although there are a few exceptions but that's what they are. Everybody knows what are good or bad lifestyles and habits, so there is no need to reiterate the extremely familiar basic things. I mean, can you find one person in civilized world who doesn't know that exercise is beneficial for the body and smoking is bad?

What I want to emphasize is the principle of *compounding*; it will not harm to have an occasional beer, but it's very difficult to stay within the limits of maximum allowed daily alcohol intake. If you have begun working out, that's great but how long are you going to continue? People say "do what you love and love what you do", but what if you drink all day and love it too?

One thing must be very clear, life's habits are not a day trade but they are equity. It doesn't matter if you have run ten miles a day for a month and then for the ensuing 11 months you do nothing.

Embracing healthy lifestyles is all you can do and it's something that you must and the best time to start healthy habits is before you turn this page. The problem is we wait and then we turn the page and don't change our bad habits still. There is no time like now and this time will lay the foundation for the rest of your life. In life there are only possibilities, there are no guarantees; everything is about a chance and the power to influence these chances is in your hands. So, you are not powerless and have command over your destiny because you can always influence your possibilities.

"Prevention is better than cure", no matter how many times I come across this line it never gets old. For cancers it is the Holy Grail, at least for me. To find the panacea will be a great discovery but the more impactful discoveries are related to prevention. It is not possible to include every preventive strategy in this book, it will be a subject of a different book; what I can say definitely is that everybody knows about the most important preventive strategies and yet most people fail to implement those. I am not an expert of human behaviour, so I will not dwell on how it so happens that people continue harmful practices and don't apply healthy changes to their lifestyles. It is information enough for me that such is the case.

I am always counselling *patients* about the preventive measures that they can take to help them recover and it is especially more important for the long-term survivors because they have a higher propensity for developing new cancers, which are called "second primaries". The diagnosis of cancer is a life changing event for the patient and it almost instantaneously puts everything in perspective for the patient. They may realise it later on, but I can see it in their eyes that something inside them has profoundly and irreversibly changed. Every action they take after the diagnosis has a whole new meaning, so I find it easier to persuade the *patients* to quit their bad habits and adopt healthy lifestyle. As far as people of good health are concerned, most of them take everything for granted until it is too late.

I have often heard people claiming that they know somebody who developed lung cancer even though he never smoked. While another person they know has been drinking a bottle of whiskey everyday and smoking like a chimney for past fifty years and is still hail and hearty. Let's look at it from another point of view; say you have two friends, one always stops at a red traffic light and the other one never stops and imagine that the friend who always follows the rules of traffic gets in an accident and gets badly injured, while the other one who always runs red lights and drives in the most rash way you can imagine, never even has a scratch throughout his life. What is the moral of the story? The fact is that there is no moral of this story, because a happenstance cannot be taken as evidence and guidance.

It is common sense that if you don't look before you cross the road then you are more likely to get hit but does this mean that you *will* get hit? Or if you always look before you cross, you will *never* get hit? These are just probabilities and probability is mathematics. Everyone knows that smoking is bad, exercises is good, unsafe sex is bad, extended exposure to sun is bad, obesity is bad, exercise is good, vegetables are good, processed foods are bad, healthy sleep is good etc. So now the question is not that there is a lack of awareness, there is plenty. The problem lies in execution. I too once was in grasp of some bad habits but when I realised that I am a person of value and my goal is bigger than me, which is to serve and heal people through my best efforts, my bad habits just disappeared. You can get rid of all your bad habits right now, and for that there is more help available today than there was ever.

With this we will move on to the next chapter, the causes (etiologies) of cancers.

CHAPTER 4
ETIOLOGY

There are some causes of cancer which are simply out of our control, factors like ageing and genetic diseases are not something we can control yet. It is a fact that cancer is a disease of the elderly, most of the cancers have their median ages of onset after the sixth decade of life. So many things change in our bodies, ultimately weakening our defence systems enough to cause cancer. Ageing as a risk factor is not something which we can control.

Genetic predisposition that makes a person more likely to develop cancer is also not modifiable. We can recognise some of the hereditary cancer symptoms and be more alert to diagnose the cancers at the earliest stages in such individuals. We can't yet genetically modify a person so that the cancer never develops, although we do know that the pattern of development of such cancers are different in these individuals, which we can use to predict the potential sites and take measures to timely diagnosis and treat them.

There are herculean feats that we have to perform if we are trying to accomplish massive success and then there are a few life situations, where to get the highest results we just have to *not* do anything. The number one reason for preventable cancer incidence is tobacco and all anybody has to prevent tobacco related cancers from ever happening is put that cigarette out or better yet never to pick it up in the first place. This holds true for other tobacco products also. Now we can all argue and start teaching each other lessons of history and psychology of human behaviour; but at the end of the day, it is a stupid act of putting a burning stick in our mouths and sucking on poisonous smoke that we have to stop.

The mechanisms by which tobacco causes cancer are operative at a genetic level and the carcinogens (mostly amines) damage the DNA. Mutations start to accumulate and there are many studies that interestingly show that many mutations occur by smoking a *single* cigarette. These mutations are repaired by our immune system and corrective mechanisms, but then as smoking quantity and time duration increases, coupled with the genetic makeup of an individual, which is unique in its interaction with these mutations, one thing leads to another and the process snowballs. Soon key regulatory repairing mechanics get affected and cancer arises.

As we have already discussed, cancer usually becomes detectable when it weighs about a gram and has a billion cells, so the cancer which has surfaced today, has been developing for many months or years. Tobacco smoking or consumption in any form has a cumulative effect. A concept of *pack-year* is often used to describe how much theoretical risk a given person has based on his smoking habits. The calculation goes like this, each pack of cigarettes has 20 cigarettes and if you smoke 20 cigarettes a day then you smoke one pack a day, so that is your average daily packs of cigarettes and then you multiply it by the number of years that you have been smoking cigarettes in such numbers, to give your *pack-year*. So, suppose you have been smoking 30 cigarettes a day then the number of packs you are smoking everyday is 1.5 packs and you have been smoking for 20 years, so we will multiply 1.5 with 20, giving 30 *pack-year*. There are charts and online tools available for this calculation and based on other risk factors a prediction can be made for the development of lung cancer in you.

This is significant, because if you meet certain criteria, then you may be eligible for *screening* for lung cancer with annual low dose CT scan. Another important fact is that if you are an active smoker and quit today, then in 15 years the risks associated with smoking greatly diminish, sometimes coming back to never-smoker levels. Passive smoking has been proven dangerous and the awareness in this regard has led to many laws being implemented throughout the world.

There is no lowest limit of *safe* tobacco consumption and everything lies on a curve of probabilities. Recently *vaping* has picked up pace and I have one answer to any queries or controversies: why smoke in any form? Have we run out of all the other things to do? There is infinite amount of exciting work always remaining to be taken care of, why not do that, instead of finding newer ways to poison ourselves?

Another known cause of cancer is viruses. Certain viruses apart from their natural course of causing their specific illnesses in humans, get one step further. What happens is that the genetic material of the virus gets integrated with the genetic material of the host and certain key regulatory mechanisms get affected, leading to development of cancer. This is not only insightful from a scientific perspective but also from a preventive or therapeutic one. We can learn much about the developmental models of cancer and utilise the knowledge to understand other cancers. There are recommendations from international organisations for HPV (papillomavirus) vaccination. HPV is a major cause of cancer of cervix, along with anogenital and oropharyngeal cancers; vaccination against this virus when given in certain age groups as per expert recommendations, has led to dramatic fall in the incidence of cervical cancer.

The discovery of association between HPV and cervix cancer was Nobel prize winning one and the resulting practical applications in form of vaccines have saved millions of lives. Other viruses like polyoma, Epstein-Barr, kaposi, retroviruses (eg, HIV) and hepatitis viruses lead to specific types of malignancies. Describing these associations in detail will lead to unnecessary prolongation of this chapter, the highlight is that some cancers have viral etiology. The prevention and treatment of these can lead to excellent outcomes on a mass level. Immunization against HPV and hepatitis viruses, and therapies directed to most of these viruses are in our arsenal and others are in development.

Third well known etiology is inflammation. Inflammation is the complex biological response of the body to irritation, injury or infection. The topic of inflammation is extremely complex and it is central to almost all other etiologies that lead to cancer development. Inflammation plays a role in every way of cancer development and targeting it, especially the NF kappa-beta pathway, using various targeted therapies has lead to clinical benefits.

Chemical factors are the fourth etiology. The list of chemicals related to carcinogenesis is very long but by understanding a few examples we can get to know the topic. Tobacco smoke is a chemical mixture, which we have already discussed. You must have heard about asbestosis; asbestos is a chemical used in many industries like cables, mining, shipyards etc. It has been known to cause many types of cancers, especially mesothelioma and lung cancer. There are many cancer with strong association with certain chemicals, knowledge of which leads not only to effective policy making for general population and industry workers but also to better understanding of carcinogenesis.

Lung cancer has been associated with many agents like tobacco smoke, asbestos, arsenic, coal tar and pitch, diesel exhaust, carbide powder etc; oral cavity cancer can be caused by tobacco smoke, alcohol, nickel compounds, betel quid; liver cancer by alcohol, tobacco, aflatoxin, vinyl chloride; cadmium has been linked to prostate cancer; benzene can cause leukemias and there are many drugs that are known causes of certain cancers. Lately, aristolochic acid has been used as a model to study urothelial cancer development. Effective understanding of the substances that you are putting in and on your body, as well as those present in your home and work environment is crucial, as the effects of these are cumulative. A little knowledge goes a long way in dealing with things of compounding nature. Awareness is key.

Physical factors are the fifth etiology. Ionizing radiation (nuclear fallout) is an infamous cause of many types of cancers and especially blood cancers. Ultraviolet light exposure is directly linked to skin cancer. Asbestosis can act both as physical and chemical factor. Radon gas present in households is a cause of lung cancer. Lately, there has been much debate about association between electromagnetic fields generated by wireless technology and cancer; although I am not an expert on research regarding this issue but I would like to advise my reader to exercise common sense. Why use something more than necessary? Water is essential for life but drinking extreme amounts of water will lead to water intoxication, electrolyte imbalance and other serious complications; in the same way technology has also become essential for modern life and it's a fact that its rate of progression is only going to accelerate, with more and more kinds of advanced technologies making ways into our lives. We can't change that, but *we* can change *ourselves* and use technology as safely and as sparingly as possible. This is my philosophy, *least of a necessary evil is the best.*

The subject of the sixth factor, diet, is one of the most controversial ones. There are so many conflicting hypothesis, and myths are plenty. Recently there have been major *setbacks* in *traditional* risk factors for other diseases; for example, the case of cholesterol and its association with diseases. Once saturated fats and cholesterol were thought to be our worst enemy and now there are diet plans, which are considered the most healthy ones, major components of which are saturated fats. So, everything is in a mix. The answer to most of the questions that my patient pose are very guarded, most of the times I give answers like: *"we don't know decisively, there is not enough data, I can't recommend for it or against it, studies have not shown a clear association"*, etc. So my patients are often confused about what to follow and what to avoid.

It is estimated that up to 35% of cancers are linked to dietary factors and it makes sense too, because we consume foods everyday, so cumulative effect is there at its fullest. But at the same time it's hard to pinpoint the healthy versus unhealthy dietary factors because the type of proof that we need to establish a theory is randomised controlled trial, and these are very difficult to perform for dietary factors. Often very long term follow-up is needed, there are endless confounding factors and, this is the most troubling part, we don't know essentially what we are looking for.

For the sake of giving out my take on these factors, I will be making generalizations here. It is advised to not blindly follow the following writing, nor to follow any other advise that you have not directly discussed with your physician as well. Total calorie consumption is linked with your body weight, and obesity plays a central role in many carcinogenic processes, so it's advisable to not overeat and similarly no to be undernourished as well. Alcohol consumption in excess is dangerous and my experience with my patients and general educational program participants has been that it's nearly impossible to stay under the limit once you start. As it's just too low to follow for most of the people. When filling up a questionnaire about their alcohol usage people are often astonished by looking at their results. My advice would be to stop drinking altogether or better yet never start.

Dietary fat, especially of animal origin, has been linked to breast, colon and prostate cancer; although the data comes mostly from animal studies and concrete recommendations are hard to make. When I tell my patients that fruit and vegetable consumption has not shown to be of much benefit in cancer prevention, they have

a look of disbelief in their eyes. Although I always advise to incorporate fruits and vegetables more in diet but evidence lacks.
Same holds true for fibre, as important role have not yet been
conclusively demonstrated. On the other hand, there is red meat;
which has been given category 1 carcinogenic status, although
with great controversy. There are so many other factors at play
here, as far as scientific guidelines are concerned, red meats are
labelled as carcinogens; but I personally would like to see more
data and studies.

Vitamin D has been found to be beneficial in colon cancer prevention, not so much in other cancers. Carotenoids and sel-
enium supplementation has famously increased cancer rates in
trials and it was a real eye-opener. Nothing conclusively can be
said about soy products and carbohydrates. On a different note,
many interesting studies are out there. Like a study linking eating
French fries during childhood with breast cancer and higher than
normal birth weight with leukaemia, but these lead nowhere as
it's impossible to remove the confounding factors. My rule of
thumb advices are, caloric balance and maintenance of healthy
body weight and muscle mass. Absolutely no tobacco consumption in any form and no excess consumption of alcohol. Consumption of a diet with high fruits and vegetables content. All
the rest is as you wish to choose; discuss with your physician or
nutritional expert and then decide for yourself and please don't
heed to fads, because at the end of the day, you are responsible for
yourself.

Eighth factor is obesity and physical inactivity. There is no need
to go on and on about it; say no to obesity and become physically
active to whatever extent you can, that is the only strategy.

CHAPTER 5
CANCER PREVENTION AND SCREENING

C ancer prevention, as a subject, is more valuable for the welfare of society than developing new therapies; because no matter how hard we try, and even succeed, in developing more and more cancer therapies, these will never be enough because cancer can always undergo mutation and it follows the principles of Darwinian evolution. One therapy may succeed or fail, but ultimately many patients would still suffer. So, the best way to fight cancer is to prevent it from ever happening and the second best way is to detect it as early as possible by *screening.*

Most of the infections in hospitals and in communities can be prevented by proper hand washing. Is this the only reason for infection? If we hand wash properly will there be no infections in the hospitals? No, that's not the case. There will still be many infections requiring other measures for their prevention, but the majority will be prevented, so we must implement this routine with utmost discipline. In the same way, if one factor, tobacco, can be just removed from society, cancer incidence will plummet astonishingly. Smoking status is considered a *vital sign* that has to be recorded at every visit to the hospital, just like blood pressure. At least it's what I practice and it does create a huge impact in understanding patterns of tobacco epidemic and counselling people. Does this mean that tobacco is the only cause or only smokers develop lung cancer? It's not like that but it's the *biggest* factor.

We must understand that tobacco has a highly addictive substance *nicotine* in it, which has clearly demonstrable neuropsychological effects. So, instead of stigmatising ourselves or others, we should try to find the solution. There are three ways to quit smoking: with the help of a counsellor, nicotine replacement therapy and with medications. Of course, these are for those who can't do it by themselves. So please ask for help, there are support programs available. Ghastly images are displayed on the packs of cigarettes and other tobacco products in many countries and I don't think in this day and age, anybody is unaware of the ill-effects of tobacco but clearly something is off. Ask for help, please.

Another important issue is continued tobacco use in a cancer patient. Some patients quit right then and there, when they come to know about the diagnosis; but in other patients an entirely different thought process arises. They feel like now the end has come, so what does it matter if they continue to smoke? It matters in three important ways: one, that it increases the chances of developing another cancer different from the one present, after successfully completing the course of treatment for present cancer; two, it increases the toxicity associated with treatment and can even decrease the effects of treatment thereby diminishing the chances of cure and three, it breaks down the morale of the patient because, think about it, patients can smoke after being diagnosed with cancer only if they have given up hope.

Nicotine is a very treacherous substance, it acts on certain areas in brain and makes the smoker feel protected and safe, that's why people smoke when they are stressed. It makes them feel *safe and in control* and when somebody develops cancer, it is one of the most psychologically traumatic events. Nicotine makes the cancer patients feel somewhat safe in the face of grave danger; at the same time patients know that this is the behaviour that gave rise to the cancer in the first place. Resultant psychological turmoil can be impossible to handle, but plenty of help is available and always ask for it.

Another preventive strategy is surgery. In certain high risk genetic conditions there is enough data to perform such surgeries. People at high risk for breast cancer, gastric cancer, ovarian, endometrial, colon and certain endocrine cancers can benefit from this strategy. If you have family history of any cancer, it's best to discuss with your doctor about how to proceed. Tests are available for general population, but should always be undertaken with help of experts.

Chemoprevention, another preventive strategy, is the use of range of interventions from drugs to isolated dietary components to whole diet modulation to block, reverse or prevent the development of invasive cancers. This topic in itself is for another book, but I can summarise it for my readers for some insight.

One thing is for sure that there is clear evidence *against* using nutritional supplements for cancer prevention as in some trials the risk actually increased and in most others, there was no benefit at all. So if you are not deficient in some nutrient, supplementation is not to be considered. A good wholesome diet is all that you need.

Anti-inflammatory drugs, mainly aspirin, have showed regression of colonic polyps in affected individuals and it may have some benefit in prevention of colorectal cancers, but high quality data is lacking for recommending it to general population; also, given the ten or more years of latency between developing a polyp and its transformation into cancer, makes it unlikely that such a trial will take place.

There are epigenetic targeting agents like tamoxifen for breast cancer along with other such medicines, these are recommended in certain populations and the results are fruitful, but take care to discuss all the pros and cons with your physician. Finasteride and dutasteride prevent or delay carcinogenesis progression in prostate but higher grade lesions occur at the same rate and there has been no clear demonstrable mortality benefits. Statins, bisphosphonates, metformin and omega-3 fatty acids have been tried with mixed results.

Another strategy is to use anti-infectives, like in cases of Helicobacter pylori bacterial infection, which affects 50% of world population. It leads to gastric cancers, the discovery of this association was a Nobel prize winning one. In areas of widespread incidence of H. pylori, mass eradication programmes have been used with some success. But this bacteria has protective effects for esophageal cancer, so it remains a question requiring further research.

At the end of such discussions with people, I find them puzzled. There is no need to be so, the key take home messages are no tobacco, no or limited alcohol consumption, maintaining healthy body weight and consulting your doctor for any preventive strategies that may be useful in your particular case.

The next best thing to prevention of cancer, is to detect it at the earliest stages, when chances of cure are the most. Cancer screening refers to a test or examination performed on an asymptomatic individual. It means certain tests should be undertaken by *everybody* in a specifically defined population; only then meaningful outcomes can be expected on mass level.

Some cancers are easily detected in early stages, like the cancer involving vocal cords will lead to hoarseness of voice at early stages most of the times; on the other hand there are cancers which become apparent when they are fairly advanced and often incurable. Then screening sounds like a very good idea because majority of cancers are not symptomatic till they are advanced, but there is a catch. If a screening test shows *something* out of the ordinary, what is to be done? Suppose a forty year old lady, who sometimes smokes, comes to your office and you order a screening chest CT scan and there is a two centimetres large nodule in the middle lobe of her right lung, what is to be done next? The problem lies not in the detection but in further course of action.

Most of the abnormalities picked up on a screening test will either never progress or are not cancerous or even resolve on their own, and the intervention and investigations required to confirm their nature pose a significant risk for the health of the individual.

Coming to the point, I recommend these following cancer screening tests in my practice: every women over 40 years should undergo screening for breast cancer, every women over 21 years and up to 65 years should undergo screening for cervix cancer, everyone over 50 years and up to 75 years (sometimes up to 85 years) should undergo screening for colorectal cancer, everyone between 55 to 74 years of age with a 30 or more *pack-year* of smoking history should undergo lung cancer screening with low dose CT scans and starting at age of 50 years, prostate cancer screening should be considered in men.

There are many nuances and subtle variations for an individual situation, like if there is strong family history, some genetic predisposition in the family or the individual then the actual tests and age limits will be different, as will be the interval between the tests. For other cancers like ovarian cancer, skin cancer etc, I personally don't recommend the screening tests; as the results of the trials are not very impactful and the interventions, which are used to prove the nature of the findings upon these tests, may even do harm.

But it's all dependent on your particular situation and consulting with your physician should be the only way forward. Sometimes people ask me if there is a battery of tests that *everybody* should go through to detect all the cancers that may or may not arise? As an answer, I always assess the individual sitting in front of me, take a thorough history, perform a physical examination and then re-

commend tests, if that person meets the criteria set by international guidelines. To my readers my simple answer is: discuss it
with your doctor.

CHAPTER 6

DIAGNOSTIC METHODS: IMAGING

This is not a textbook, nor it is my intention to make this book academic and boring to my reader, although I can assure you that the academic studies of cancers are one of the most exciting materials to read.

History of the present complaints and physical examination are irreplaceable and many times more valuable than the most advanced tools medicine has to offer. And more importantly the physical examination builds a bond between patient and the doctor. A *funeral* may have been performed by AMA for physical examination, but a thorough physical examination is a part of my practice and it always will be.

Everything in medical science is an art to some degree and physical examination is one of the major and toughest of these arts to master, but it has its own limitations. So, further advances have been made by science for the diagnosis and to give more objective outcomes, which are less observer dependent.

Imaging studies like X-ray, mammogram, ultrasound, CT scan, MRI scan and PET scan etc have each something to offer. There is not a single *know it all* method which can be applied to every patient with the perfect result every time. For example, CT scan may not be able to fully evaluate a liver lesion and ultrasound is sometimes more helpful although it is far less expensive.

Then there are various "scopies", like upper GI endoscopy, colonoscopy, bronchoscopy, laryngoscopy and more. Scopies help us directly visualise the hollow structures of our bodies. There are many other less frequently used imaging modalities as well.

There has been many considerable debates about the proper usage of diagnostic imaging modalities; and the over and under usage of the same. Sometimes these can do more harm than good, like the lung cancer screening trials found out that most of the abnormalities detected on low dose CT scans of smokers were actually not significant and lead to unnecessary interventions.

Everything has to be looked into with scientific perspective because if the doctor finds something upon an imaging study then something must be done, both to dispel any suspicion of cancer and to allay the anxiety of the patient.

Judicious use of these immensely powerful and informative tools can't be emphasised enough. Not only for the false positive findings, but the financial burden and the carcinogenicity associated with the radiation, which is a part of most of these modalities.

In practice many patients come to me and ask for a whole body PET-CT scan, just because they think they have cancer and they want to get rid of these suspicions. What essentially happens in some of these patients is that some lesions are detected of undetermined significance and at sites, that are dangerous to access. So, I observe such patients with serial scanning, resulting in both patients' psychological turmoil and financial burden, not to mention danger to their health.

Many guidelines throughout the world have been published and their summarise nicely, what's to be done and when and how. It is always wise to ask your doctor about any screening programs which may benefit you. Each individual has unique risk factors and in my opinion consultation with your physician about the appropriate strategy tailored to you is very important. And if you are a candidate for screening, then the approved screening modalities have more benefits than risk, as established by a plethora of published evidence. Then of course, the potential risks associated with these techniques can be taken in order to obtain the benefits associated with that screening program.

CHAPTER 7

DIAGNOSTIC METHODS: TISSUE DIAGNOSIS

Barring a very few exceptions, cancer diagnosis requires histological or cytological proof, that means that we must be able to *see* the cancerous cells through our eyes to finalize the diagnosis. Before getting in details, let's revise some of the queries that I have in my practice, the most common ones are: *"will it be painful*?", many ask *"is it a must to do a biopsy?"*, some of my patients ask that if their biopsy or cytology report comes back negative for cancer, will it mean they don't have cancer, but above all these queries there is one very popular question that keeps popping up: *"will it **spread** my cancer"*?

We must understand that cancer is a histological or cytopathological diagnosis, it requires proof not only to diagnose it but to decide which type of therapy is to be given; in other words it's imperative to obtain a proper diagnosis for a scientific management of cancer. We just can't say that a lamp is cancerous based on other diagnostics. The procedure used for obtaining tissue may be painful, it may give false negative results, sometimes equivocal results as well and there are a set of protocols in place which are results of decades of medical research to perform such procedures.

As far as spreading of cancers is concerned, the potential infinitesimally small risk of such an occurrence is far too low compared to the apparent benefits of these procedures. Of course, there are some cancers like renal cell carcinoma, hepatocellular cancer and choriocarcinoma among others, which sometimes don't require a tissue specimen and if such is the case the doctor will inform you of the same.

There are risks involved with any procedure, but it is through the analysis of data we reach at the conclusion as to what has to be done in face of danger. After cytology, biopsy or any other such procedure is performed, the cancer cells are visualized and pathologists report the type of cancer along with its subtype and many other subtle but very important features. In case of doubt, immunohistochemistry stains (IHC) or genetic tests among other tests, are used as needed. In this way, a final diagnosis is reached, based on that final diagnosis the existing worldwide accepted guidelines for that particular type of cancer are followed.

To summarise, most of the times pathological diagnosis is where the treatment of cancer begins; so please let go of any fears or misconceptions you may have about the procedures of obtaining samples of cancer; remember that the risk is almost zero and the benefits of a diagnosis are hundred percent.

CHAPTER 8
STAGING

I work in a charitable hospital in my home state, as my aspiration always was to give back to the society. The least I can do is to help the people I know the most, and who are in need of help. There are people coming to my office from all walks of life, some are highly educated, while others are utterly illiterate; but one question they all have when it comes to their diagnosis: *"what is the stage of my cancer?"*

Due to awareness campaigns, this word *"stage"*, is known to everyone and it is one of the most powerful statements about cancer that a doctor can make. So, we ought to understand what stage actually means. If cancer is a fire, then the extent to which the fire has spread is the *stage* and the lesser the stage, the easier it is to control the cancer, just as it is for a fire. Suppose the fire has just started in the corner of the room that you are sitting in now, if you immediately put it out, how much would be the damage? It would be minimal and more importantly nothing else will be damaged; but then the fire can get so out of control, if no intervention is done on appropriate time, that it can destroy the entire building beyond salvage.

There are many cancer staging systems and many cancers have their own staging systems, which are applicable to only those cancers. Most of the cancers are staged by American Joint Committee on Cancer (AJCC) staging system, which is otherwise known as TNM staging. T for tumor, N for nodes and M for metastasis. AJCC regularly updates their staging system. The staging systems are not just informative about the extent to which cancer has spread but also are essential for effective decision making and policy making. The details are overwhelming but to simplify, if the tumor is still within the organ from which it originated it is generally stage one or two, if it has spread to nodes then it is stage three, if it has spread to adjacent organs then it can be stage three or four and if it has spread to other areas of the body, it is stage four. I want to emphasize that it is an *extreme* oversimplification and exceptions are many.

Staging is an exercise tailored to the particular cancer and patient, to determine the best treatment strategy. Does it mean that if you are stage one then you will *definitely* get cured and if you are stage four then there are no chances of cure? It is not the case, the survival data corresponding to stages are just probabilities. An individual can either get one hundred percent cured or not at all. Staging is for treatment decisions, policy making, trial designing and uniform implementation of effective treatments but it is definitely not for patients to decide at what stage they will give up.

I have seen many stage one patients suffer an ill fate and stage four patients getting miraculously cured. Remember, if the chances of survival are as low as 10%, they are still better than 0% and if the chances of death are 1% and the patient dies; then, for that patient mortality rate is hundred percent. Staging is not to be intimidated of, it's just a number and each person is unique. So, whatever you do, please don't decide on your own when it is too late. It's the responsibility of the treating doctor to inform you about all the aspects and treatment options, which are best suited for your particular condition.

CHAPTER 9
TREATMENT: GENERAL PRINCIPLES

I t is hard to summarize even the basic principles of cancer management, but we will try to have an overview of what means what in cancer. The first principle of cancer treatment is *"primum non nocere";* meaning first, to do no harm. The second principle is *"hasten to help".* What these principles essentially mean is that cancer in itself is a deadly disease and quiet debilitating as well; and the therapies required for cancer are often very aggressive and morbid themselves. So, we must strike a balance between the adverse effects and loss of functionality from these therapies, and the outcomes we are expecting by their usage.

Sometimes it is simply not possible to cure cancer. In these instances, our primary aim shifts to prolongation of life, reducing the adverse effects caused by therapy and most importantly, improving the quality of life. On the other hand, if the cancer is in a curable stage then we have to undertake radical measures like amputations, removal of whole organs, intensive chemotherapy regimens or extended radiotherapy schedules; because we are trying to cure the patient for life and we should not leave any chance for the cancer cells to remain in the body and proliferate again. But this too we have to undertake in a way which is least harmful for the patient, in this way we are *first doing no harm and then hastening to help.*

There are three modalities of cancer treatment: surgery, radiation therapy and chemotherapy. Most of the blood related (hematological) cancers are treated by chemotherapy and some of them may require stem cell transplant. There is not much role of surgery and radiation therapy in management of these cancers.

On the other hand, *solid cancers* are managed according to their stage. When they are in the earliest stages, the most appropriate and first treatment is often surgery. Surgery is curative alone in certain settings but most of the time some form of therapy is required after surgery like chemo, radiation or a combination of both. These therapies, which we are giving after surgery are known as *adjuvant therapy.*

If however, the cancer is localized but cannot be resected or the surgery required to remove such extensive disease will be excessively morbid, then chemo, radiation or both can be used before surgery to make it possible and less morbid; these therapies are then known as *neoadjuvant therapies.*

In some circumstances, when radiation can give similar cure rates compared to surgery and is way less morbid, then it can be used as the primary treatment modality instead of surgery.

Apart from a few exceptions like choriocarcinoma, chemotherapy is not able to cure a solid malignancy on its own; although in advanced stage and metastatic malignancies, chemotherapy is often the only resort. Combinations of chemotherapies, single-agent chemotherapy, targeted therapy, immunotherapy are used in advanced and metastatic settings to improve the quality of life and increase the lifespan of the patient. In such metastatic cases surgery and radiation have their limited roles, mostly in palliative settings.

The take home message I want to give to my readers is: in most of the cases all three modalities of cancer treatment are used. In fact, by governmental regulations in many countries, a cancer hospital must have a *tumor board;* which is constituted by doctors from all three treating specialties as well as pathologists, radiologists and other doctors too, when needed. So you should try to get a *tumor board opinion* always and if possible meet other doctors of the tumor board as well.

CHAPTER 10
SURGERY

I t is the most ancient and time-tested form of cancer treatment. From the earliest available manuscripts to the latest research papers, the importance of surgery in treatment of cancer is unquestionably paramount. The premise is simple: remove the diseased tissue. Surgery can be open, laparoscopic or robotic depending on the disease site and guidelines.

The extent of surgery is determined by the disease, its site, size and various other factors. Every effort is made to maximize the oncological outcome while maintaining function and minimising morbidity. Sometimes surgery can be done at the very outset and in some instances, it is done after some form of other therapy like chemo, radiation or a combination of both.

The principles of oncology is *first do no harm* and then *hasten to help*. Every form of cancer treatment causes a unique challenge to the treating doctor, as all cancer treatments are essentially *harming* the patient in some way. For instance, an osteosarcoma of lower end of the femur may require amputation of the leg. This will be treating the patient but with inherent harm involved, as the patient is losing a limb. So, while surgery is the most curative and best possible option till date for almost all of the solid cancers, it should be contemplated with the concept of *first no harm*. That is why leaving a few exceptions, almost all cancers require some form of adjuvant (after surgery) and/or neoadjuvant (before surgery) treatment to maximize upon the surgical outcomes while minimising the extent of surgery that may otherwise be required, as may be the case.

I find it hard to explain to the patient why such radical surgery is needed and even if they are willing to undergo such surgery, why chemo or radiation is still needed. I have enormous respect for oncosurgeons, they have to undergo extensive training and cancer surgery is unlike any other surgery; the sheer complexity and depth of understanding needed is staggering.

I have one message for my readers that if surgery can be done then it has to be done and that too as soon as possible. It can be disastrous to wait and squander time, as many of the common malignancies have doubling times of around 3 to 4 weeks.

That being said, it is equally important to remember that cancer is a systemic disease, meaning that it involves the whole body and not just the site to which it is seemingly confined. If there is a breast lump of 2 cm and rest of the body has no visible disease then too the treatment is almost always multimodality, meaning that chemo and radiation are needed. Of course there are exceptions, like breast cancers with favourable OncotypeDX or other such assays, but they are not the rule.

We otherwise have come a long way from the heroic Halstedian approach to more and more conservative surgery and incorporating other modalities at every step. Science of cancer is evolving, but today the most definitive answer to almost all of the solid tumors is surgery. It's always wise to act promptly when action is needed and when it comes to cancer treatment, attack is the best defence. Once cancer is diagnosed, it's of no use to find non-scientific remedies and we must go for cure; and if possible and appropriate, for surgery, no matter how radical it will be.

CHAPTER 11
RADIATION THERAPY

Radioactive sources, like cobalt, emit energy in form of radiation; scientists have harnessed this power to kill cancer cells. Radioactive source is kept in a chamber, it keeps on emitting radiation continuously based on principles of radioactive decay and this energy is directed via a machine to the cancerous areas of the patient. This process is made precise by software programs and clinical data application based on many factors.

Nowadays newer technology has replaced radioactive source based therapies. These newer therapies are linear accelerators, proton beam, carbon ion etc. In linear accelerator machines, high energy electrical input generates megavolt rays, which are guided by complex computer algorithms to deliver precise doses. Proton beam machines are also popping up on the world map, they have a unique energy distribution property (Bragg peak), which leads to lesser injury to normal tissue.

Radiation therapy is the most versatile cancer treatment approach. It can ablate a very small lesion deep inside the most sensitive areas of the brain, as well as cover very large areas, some times as much as half or whole, of the body. This modality is curative for many cancers alone and an integral part of treatment of many others. For instance, cancer of vocal cords (larynx) when treated with surgery will lead to loss of speech function in most of the cases, while they can be cured with radiation with preservation of speech.

People have many misconceptions about radiation therapy, like it will burn them, it will hurt them, or it can cause death; the simple fact is that it's one of the safest approach among other options and side effects are well manageable. Modern radiation delivery machines are extremely sophisticated and in fact, the biggest expense by a wide margin in setting up a cancer hospital goes to radiation department establishment.

Adverse effects related to radiation therapy are generally localised and depend on the site of treatment. Like in head and neck cancers, the toxicities are mostly ulcers (mucositis) and dryness of mouth (xerostomia). While treating lung cancers and other thoracic structures, radiation pneumonitis can result. These radiation associated toxicities are well manageable.

To understand a few technicalities, there are many types of radiation techniques but simply put they are external beam radiation, during which the patient lies on a cot under the machine; and internal, when the source of radiation is placed inside the body, also known as brachytherapy.

Usually the external beam settings use *fractionation* which means that the dose is first calculated considering all the known factors and then it's divided into many small fractions and given many days of a week, for a few weeks. Of course, there are many other ways, like many sessions in a single day known as *hyperfractionation* or high dose given with lesser fractions known as *hypofractionation* or maybe even in just a few sittings, using stereotactic methods known as SBRT.

Whatever is the approach, one fact I would like to convey to my readers is that radiation therapy is a real lifesaver and is much less morbid than other modalities of cancer treatment. Many times I have seen patients refusing radiation right off the bat, as they have reservations about it and when I ask them the reasons for their reservations, they aren't able to tell me anything other than some anecdotes; so, most of the time they have not even obtained the information from somebody actually treated with radiotherapy. There is no need to unnecessary worry about the myths that are in circulation. While it's true that several decades back radiotherapy technology was indeed rudimentary and ridden with myriads of adverse effects but that's no longer the case.

CHAPTER 12

CHEMOTHERAPY

At its inception, chemotherapy and especially combinations of these drugs, were considered absurd and downright harmful for the patients. It was a controversial time and it took decades for scientific community and practitioners to fully adopt those protocols.

The word *chemotherapy* translates into therapy using chemicals, for any disease. But slowly chemotherapy, as a word, has become synonymous with medicines used to treat cancer. These are molecules that have the ability to kill cancer cells. The mechanisms by which different chemo work, is a subject of another book; they can be cell cycle specific or nonspecific, targeted or conventional and they can be classified according to their molecular structures.

One common underlying activity is that all chemo somehow damage DNA of cancer cells, thus leading to their death. Chemo are unique among medicines, because they not only kill the cancerous cells but also normal cells. To understand this, let's take the example of antibiotics. Antibiotics are also *killers*, but their primary mode of action is directed towards the *prokaryotic* genetic material of bacteria, although they harm our cells too but not to a great degree because our cells are *eukaryotic*, with essential differences from bacteria.

Chemo on the other hand is killing cells that are our *own*; of course, they are damaged cells but they are derivatives of our own cells. This makes the task of eradicating these cancer cells by chemicals very difficult. On one hand, we have to kill the cancer cells which are very much alike our normal cells; and on the other hand, we have to minimize the damage caused to normal cells. This is the reason for developing toxicities from chemo.

The adverse effects of chemo most often involve rapidly dividing cells, like that of our gastrointestinal mucosa, hair follicles and bone marrow; thus leading to side effects like ulcers, diarrhea, hair loss, infection, bleeding etc. Then there are side effects like nausea, vomiting and specific side effects due to unique mode of actions of different chemo.

One fact ought to be clearly understood, *chemo has side effects.* We can minimize the incidence and reduce the severity once they happen, but side effects happen universally. With progress in oncomedicine there are many drug delivery systems available, so are targeted therapies that, as their name suggests, target specific molecules of cancer cells which minimizes the toxicity to normal cells. But even these *targeted therapies* have innumerable side effects. Even the latest development in oncology, *immunotherapy*, has toxicities, although with a different profile.

That being said, the targeted therapies available today are a blessing. Not only they are cancer cell specific and less toxic to normal tissues, but they are way better for survival outcomes as well. Targeted therapies most often are directed towards either a structure present on tumor cells, like in case of *rituximab*, which is an antibody that acts on CD20 molecules on a cancer cell and used mostly in lymphoma. Or they may target a *driver mutation*.

A *driver mutation* is the master switch for a specific cancer subset. All the mechanisms operating downstream of this master switch are very different from each other and if we stop one mechanism then another mechanism arises, due to the *plasticity* of cancer pathways, because as we know cancer cells are *alive* too and they want to survive, so they adapt. But if that master switch can be turned off, then cancer cells can't survive because the very defect due to which they originate in the first place, gets blocked. The success story of BCR-ABL directed therapies in chronic myeloid leukemia; EGFR, ALK and ROS1 directed therapies in lung cancer and many others are poof of the principle.

The process of development of these drugs is very complex and confounded by many variables. We have been able to identify the driver mutations and targets in a some cancers, but most other cancers either have no specific driver mutation but many, or they have just not been identified yet. Newer techniques like next generation sequencing (NGS) and others are unfolding newer vistas for personalized medicine and drug development. We can be certain that we can only go forward and future holds promise.

CHAPTER 13

IMMUNOTHERAPY

T here are many weapons in warfare, from knives to the biggest explosives; yet the perfect weapon is a soldier. A highly trained and skilled professional is the best of all weapons. Same holds true for cancer therapeutics and the metaphorical soldier is our own body.

It has been scientifically proven that each day thousands of lethal mutations take place in everybody, and millions of potentially cancerous cells are produced due to the inevitable defects in our genetic machinery. If left unchecked this will lead to development of many cancers in an individual, in a very short amount of time (like in genetic syndromes xeroderma pigmentosum, Fanconi's anemia etc); but as we can observe, cancers arise only in a fraction of the population.

This is made possible by the corrective mechanisms that are operating in our bodies incessantly (like TP53 gene, which is known as the *"guardian of the genome"*, it is defective is more than 50% cancers). The scope of this discussion is bewildering, so it will suffice to say that without our protective mechanisms we will all have cancer. One leading researcher recently stated that it was baffling, how *few* people develop cancer, taking in to account the scientific predictive models.

Coming back to the perfect weapon, the other modalities of cancer treatment are not so perfect. Surgery removes the cancerous part but it often results in removal of entire affected organ or other structures as well, radiation kills cancer but may damage nearby structures and chemo kills cancer cells but with collateral damage to normal cells. All this happens because the fight is between the normal *you* and the cancerous *you*.

But what if we can combine the machinery that takes care of literally thousands of mutations every day, with our knowledge of the defects or shortcomings in that machinery which cancer cells exploit to thrive? The result will be wonderful and they are. Recently awarded Nobel Prizes in medicine were for immunotherapy discovery.

What immunotherapy essentially does is that it unleashes our immune system, which cancer cells have shut down using evasive mechanisms. There is a whole chain of events that takes place, from the recognition by our immune cells that *something is off* about the cancer cells and activation of other cells and chemicals for effective killing of these defective cells. We are not introducing a *new* immune system with the immunotherapy drugs, we are just helping our already existing and very efficient immune system by removing certain chemical blocks that the cancer cells have produced for their survival, by *fooling* it. Once those chemical reactions are interrupted, the immune system recognises the cancer cells and kills them.

Of course, the modern immunotherapy is far from perfect; it has only just begun. And it is very complicated because we are trying to tweak the very fabric of life. A better array of markers for patient selection and more knowledge of other pathways involved is evolving and progress is being made every day.

It is revolutionary. I remember when I just sent stage four patients home after they failed two to three chemotherapies, and even if I continued the treatment; I knew, no improvement is to be expected; the side effects were more than the effects after many lines of chemotherapies. Now it's no longer the case. I have seen results in many cancers like lung, melanoma, kidney, head and neck, lymphoma and many others who were heavily pre-treated with many chemotherapies and they just went into remission! It's like a fairy tale but better, because it's true. Yes, it's not perfect and we have a long way to go but there is enough light at the end of the tunnel.

CHAPTER 14

ADVERSE EFFECTS

*E*very drug is a poison and every poison is a drug, it is a quote an undergraduate medical student learns in pharmacology. This is applicable to chemotherapy even more, as they have a unique task to perform. Suppose somebody has got malaria, you give them antimalarial medicine and they usually get better with minimal side effects. If somebody has got chest pain due to myocardial infarction, you do angioplasty (stenting) and they get better dramatically. What happens when someone comes for treatment of cancer and you give them chemotherapy? More often than not, they get worse for sometime, as chemo takes time to work and some to the adverse effects are pretty quick to manifest.

Chemo destroys cancerous and normal cells both, even many *targeted therapies* have innumerable side effects. People often ask me "what side effects will be there from this chemotherapy?" and I find myself in an awkward position every time when I begin to explain the side effects, from the most common ones to the rarest of rare, as nowadays not doing so can result in a lawsuit.

And with each new adverse effect they get to hear, the more and more frightened and confused they become. Now I am not saying that medicines other than chemo don't have adverse effects; in fact, if you knew all the adverse effects of paracetamol or aspirin, you will not be able to take these drugs, but the adverse effects of chemo are more intense and more common. It just never happens that chemo doesn't cause adverse effects.

These range from hair loss to death, and death is not rare. Some are life-threatening in short term, while others are late toxic effects, like leukemias developing in cancer survivors many years after treatment or sterility.

There is extensive literature on adverse events, their presentation and treatment; which basically is the study of medical oncology. The adverse effects and the certainty that the patient *will* suffer due to treatment stretches *primum non nocere* to its limits.

To my readers I have a message: when it comes to chemotherapy and its adverse effects, remember that *they will be there.* Just as you feel sore if you workout really heavy, as you feel hungry if you go on an extended fast or just as you feel sleepy after working many nights in in a row, you *will* face adverse effects if given chemotherapy. All these other activities we do to make our lives better, often result in some pain or discomfort; so in the same way chemo has its adverse effects that are part and parcel of its ability of making us better. And always remember that the oncologist is there for taking care of just that.

Giving a chemotherapy protocol is not a big deal, I call it 10% of my practice; 90% of my job is managing the adverse effects and adjusting further doses or even changing the protocol based on published guidelines and expert opinion. Don't fear because you are not alone, we are on this journey together and we shall prevail.

CHAPTER 15

PERSONALISED MEDICINE

Every cancer is unique in itself and the *patient* having that particular cancer is also unique. No two cancer patients are the same, even if their diseases are seemingly indistinguishable; this knowledge led to the concept of personalized medicine. Although in a way medicine has always been personalized, but the explosion in molecular biology and biotechnology has opened a whole new dimension.

We can now study the genetics of a patient and the cancer, which then lead us to formulate the treatment protocol that is *tailor made* for that particular patient. Nothing fits better than a tailor made apparel. Then why are we not practising this in every case? That is because the knowledge in this field is far from perfect and is barely enough in a select few cases.

All the targeted therapies and some other forms of therapies are specific to the cancers having certain similarities in their genetic makeup, although it's all too difficult to combine that small bit of cancer specific information with the whole genomic landscape of cancer and the normal genetic counterpart in the patient.

It is being practiced as much as possible with the resources that we have. The future holds promise for personalised medicine, if we continue down this path; or it can move in an entirely different direction, with use of immunotherapy like models of drug development but only time will tell. For the time being, it's always good to ask your doctor about the possibility of usage of personalised medicine in your case.

CHAPTER 16
TRANSPLANTATION

C ancer therapy sometimes requires transplantations. Most frequently it's hematopoietic stem cell transplant (HSCT) also, somewhat less accurately, known as bone marrow transplant. Liver transplants are used for liver cancer in selected cases, renal transplants are needed in a few cancers, although there are many other forms of transplants also performed but they depend on individual case by case basis.

HSCT is of two basic types, autologous and allogeneic. When patient's own stem cells are used, it's autologous and when someone else gives stem cells, it's allogeneic. Then there are umbilical cord blood transplants. For allogeneic transplants, a donor is matched against certain markers of the patient known as *"HLA matching"*. After a matched stem cell collection, some form of intense chemo is given called as *"conditioning"*, which results in *"ablation"* of patient's marrow reserves, following which the collected stem cells are infused into the patients. These new stem cells make the patient's marrow their new home, known as *"grafting"*. And then there is recovery, graft versus host and graft versus leukaemia effects or things may go south and graft may get rejected, infections may set in, there may be excessive graft versus host disease and patients may even die.

Patients often ask me about transplants and sometimes their questions are ridden with misconceptions, but that is expected. Often patients' ideas of the utility of transplants in certain situations are misplaced, like a patient of breast cancer whose cancer has metastasized to both her lungs and that too quiet extensively, asked me whether both of her lungs can be transplanted, the answer is obviously no. On the other hand high-dose chemo coupled with autologous stem cell transplant has been used as a treatment strategy in advanced breast cancer, although guidelines do not recommended it any more.

The topic of transplant is a very important one because it has something to offer, that other modalities often fail to offer in certain scenarios: cure. If you undergo a hematopoietic stem cell transplant in a condition in which it's indicated, then it does not guarantee cure; but it gives hope of obtaining it, which otherwise may not be possible. In many solid tumors like germ cell tumor, HSCT is performed when all else has failed and a fair number of patients are cured.

Overall, transplants are rigorous processes and it can be overwhelming to learn about even the basic minimum facts. To my understanding the most confusing part of my dialogue with the cancer patients is the expected survival after transplant and the risk of mortality related to transplant also known as transplant related motility or TRM. For instance, a patient of acute myeloid leukaemia, whose leukaemia had relapsed after first course of chemo was sitting across me and I was explaining to him about the process of transplantation. He was 32 years old, he understood every aspect of the process itself quite readily. Then at the end of the conversation he said that he was ready to undergo this procedure because it would cure him. It was then very difficult for him to hear when I told him that the chances of cure are very less and, in fact, chances of dying due to the procedure were greater than the cure rate in his particular case.

Transplantation is a tremendous effort, which in expert hands can lead to miraculous recoveries, but it is not a guaranteed cure; although it's often the best option when used in its specific settings. Patient must undergo these procedures for best chances of getting cured, if the doctors and guidelines recommend so.

CHAPTER 17

PAIN

While treating my patients, I am most concerned about pain. I believe it is a basic human right to be free of pain. Cancer pain comes in many different forms like bony pain, neuropathic pain, visceral pain etc. Pain management has become a specialised branch of medicine with a great variety of drugs and interventions available.

Pain management must be included with prime importance at every step of cancer management and unlike other modalities of treatment which are utilised less and less as the disease becomes more and more advanced; the pain management therapies must be used increasingly, as needed, till the end of life in my opinion. Cancer patients have the right to live, and die, free of pain.

What I have seen in practice though, is far less aggressive approach is taken towards pain management. I consider it your right to ask your doctor to do whatever it takes to make sure you are pain free. To me, there is no *acceptable* level of pain, it just shouldn't be there. Generally the patients afflicted most with cancer induced pain are those of advanced stages and while every cancer physician contemplates the nuances and subtleties of different cancer directed therapies, it is not often the case when it comes to pain management.

"*WHO ladder*" is often used, which is a guideline of the sequences of pain medicines available, but it often turns out to be a ladder reaching nowhere due to lack of its proper implementation, especially in developing world. The sequence of drugs is not followed properly; overprescribing is done in less severe pain, under prescribing is often there in those with uncontrolled pain; also neurolysis and radiation often are not rationally used. Measures should be taken proactively.

When I explain their diagnosis and prognosis to my patients; they have, more often than not, acceptance of the terminal nature of their illness, they listen patiently to the treatment options and are not afraid to make a decision but one fear, which according to at least what I have seen in my practice, greater than that of death is of pain.

At the end stages of life, patients and their relatives are most concerned about the pain that the patient might have to endure and they always request me to make sure that pain is not there. They often accept death but never pain. I would request my readers to always ask your doctor, as many times as needed, to do something about pain, if you are in any and to explore more options if pain is not alleviated; cancer-related pain is just not acceptable.

CHAPTER 18

STATISTICAL METHODS IN CANCER

A t every step of cancer treatment, I have to tell patients about the benefits of the therapy that I am planning to give. Every recommended cancer treatment has a degree of benefit that outweighs the risks, but what is this benefit in actuality?

If I am planning to remove the appendix in a case of appendicitis, then I will not be telling the patient much about the anticipated benefit as it's quite apparent, and most of my counselling will be about the harm the procedure potentially has. The treatment of cancer is unique among medical sciences as the outcomes are sometimes hard to understand.

An example of benefit is increase in *progression free survival* by a drug but not in *overall survival*; so what this means is the time period in which the disease doesn't progress increases thus patients enjoy a life without disease progression for that period of time, but the actual lifetime of the patient is not increased. **The end points of cancer treatment are both difficult to understand and sometimes frustrating.**

Almost all of the patients in my practice have to pay from their pockets for treatment and when I tell them that they have got a certain stage four malignancy and they are best treated with immunotherapy, if it is recommended for that cancer; they ask about the price of such a treatment and upon hearing it, they often go into deep thought. I am asking them to spend all of their life savings, and maybe even more on this treatment, so naturally they expect it to work like a miracle; then I tell them about different approaches that don't use such an expensive treatment, but are not as effective. At the end of the day, they want at least some guarantee from me that they will fare better with the expensive therapy but I can't say so, I just recite the data and let them decide. But how can they?

We should understand that when it comes to cancer treatment the first and foremost thing you should ask your doctor is *overall survival benefit*, that is how much life does the treatment prolong compared to others. Overall survival is the gold standard for measuring outcomes. Like in ALK mutation positive stage four lung cancer, now the treatments with latest TKIs can prolong the life well over 4 years, so that is a big leap compared to conventional cytotoxic chemotherapies. While some other therapies, like antiangiogenic therapy in certain ovarian cancer *relapse* settings, have not led to increased overall survival but they improve progression free survival.

What I am essentially telling you is to be conscious about the outcomes you are expecting and what is the reality of the situation as a whole. *The best is not always better*, and you must take everything into account before deciding, because believe it or not *you* will have to decide, as oncologists can only provide options.

CHAPTER 19
CLINICAL TRIALS

International guidelines state that the best place for treatment of any cancer patient is ideally in a clinical trial. What it highlights is the importance of this tremendous scientific tool at our disposal.

We take many things for granted. When I tell my patients about the option of enrollment in a clinical trial, they are very sceptical; but they don't know that most of the so called "*standard and time-tested treatments*" existing today, are all and I mean *all*, are the results of clinical trials. What we call a *standard treatment* today, was very experimental just a decade ago and this has been the story throughout the history of oncology. Many of the breakthrough therapies that are so widely sought after these days, have many trials ongoing comparing even more promising treatments against them.

We must understand that clinical trials are not based on the whims of mad scientists. A trial begins as an animal study and then government sanctions them after thorough vetting. The doctors and ancillary members of the trial team take care of everything and they document every little thing; then there may be crossovers, meaning if a treatment begins to fail then patients in that "arm" of the study are switched over to the other arm. There are ethical committees overwatching everything and the levels of dedication are immense.

Many times I have read this headline in newspaper and digital media, "these many patients have died in clinical trials since such and such year." This is a shameless and ungrateful way of dealing with the only scientific method to test any hypothesis in medical sciences. People who make these claims about clinical trials being evil, are the same people who want to make the *latest drugs* available to all.

My friends, please understand that technology is not self progressive; thousands of people work day and night to make it possible, and the people who have this flame of new discovery kindling in their hearts are the most precious people, without these out of the box thinkers, civilization will stagnate. I will stress again that the only method to prove a scientific hypothesis, at least in medical sciences, is a randomised controlled trial. And these trials are not secretive, their results are out in the open, available online for anyone to read, criticize and improve upon.

So please stop demonizing clinical trials, because if it were not for clinical trials and scientific methods, cancer patients today would have been getting treated with bloodletting and bromide.

CHAPTER 20
CHILDHOOD CANCERS

As a man of science, I can tell you much about the cancers arising in childhood, there unique biology and treatment principles but that will be quite a dry read and lead nowhere to a reader without a medical background. Childhood cancer pose a significant question: *"is there more to cancer?"*

To an uninitiated person looking for *a reason* for the development of cancers, to find out the *culprit*, like a bad habit; it's very difficult to grasp cancers developing in children. We often stigmatise smokers for developing lung cancer, but what about those who never smoked and still develop lung cancer and what about children who develop cancer when they are mere toddlers?

Genetics is almost everything in cancer. Most of the pediatric cancers have an underlying genetic cause, which may be inherited or sporadic. Much research has been done in this field and has shown the distinctive genotypic patterns in many childhood malignancies. On a different note, during my post graduation days I was seeing an incessant flow of children with all sorts of cancers, in our regional cancer centre.

One question always troubled me. I wasn't much perplexed by adults developing cancers, but when a child came with acute lymphoblastic leukaemia, Wilms' tumor, retinoblastoma or any other tumor; I couldn't stop pitying the poor soul and I couldn't even imagine the suffering these little ones had to endure. One of my seniors said something to me one day that changed my perspective about that. "The child is not attaching any meaning to the diagnosis, we are." How true. Then I realised as I observed more keenly that children in our wards were not much in grief; of course, when they were in pain they cried, but they were not as much psychologically distressed as their parents or treating doctors. Of course, this is not a relief from the horrible situation these children are in, but it is enough deliverance for me from the pain I was in then.

Paediatric cancers have same oncological principles as the cancers of adults, what's different is the specialisation of doctors, which is absolutely paramount; psychological support to the parents is much more needed than the adult patients' family and the therapies are often more intensive, with long-term repercussions. Many of the childhood cancers are not bestowed uponwith the same resources by the "*big pharma*", as adult cancers. Trials are there but funding is often scarce, doctors are reluctant to treat and specialists are in such short supply that it's unthinkable, at least in resource poor settings.

Acute lymphoblastic leukaemia was once considered a revolving door of death and its successful treatment was a benchmark for future cancer research. In favorable subsets of this once uniformly deadly cancer, the cure rates exceed 90%. Similarly in other pediatric cancers, following the state-of-the-art protocols gives wonderful results.

I feel especially privileged to have the honor of treating the children, the little angels born with suffering in this world and when they actually get cured nothing can compare to that feeling; especially when they go on about their lives, have children themselves and come to you to introduce them.

CHAPTER 21

PALLIATIVE AND END OF LIFE CARE

We must do what we can, but to what end? It is a question of paramount importance to me in every area of life. Yes, I can do everything; but *why* I am doing it? That is the question which is more important to me then *how* am I going to do it, because in my view every action should have a purpose and the purpose is always in the more existential question *why*.

More often than not, I find myself in conversation with a young cancer patient, somewhere in his mid thirties or even twenties, and the disease has progressed in such a way that there remains no cure for it. This patient is going to die in the next few months; that's the truth sometimes, no matter how harsh.

Now, we must understand that medical oncology is an ocean of knowledge, in which if you dive, you never come out empty handed; there is always another line of chemo, immunotherapy or clinical trials. These situations bring the personality traits of the treating doctor to surface. While some are very aggressive and keep administering toxic chemicals in their patients' bodies till the very end. I have witnessed some patients, apparently terminally ill and approaching the end of life, having been administered intensive chemos while on mechanical ventilation.

On the other hand there are doctors who incorporate palliative care right from the beginning of treatment of advanced stage patients, while gradually transitioning them fully to palliative care team.

Palliative care has a complex definition but to simplify it we can say "it's medical treatment solely aimed at improving the quality of life of the patients". It uses all the modalities of therapy and social support to deliver the patient from his suffering.

Palliative care is not just a humanitarian approach to the terminally ill cancer patients, it has been proven in trials to improve overall survival of patients, almost to the levels attained by many modern therapeutic approaches.

Now I am not going to say that we should just focus on palliation, because that will paralyze new cancer research, as most of the new drugs developed are first tested in the terminal patients and then gradually shifted to curative and less advanced cancer settings. At the same time, it's imperative to integrate palliation in the treatment plan because the ultimate aim of any medical discovery is to reduce human suffering.

To come to another topic, it is often said that hospitals are the ivory towers of diseases. Research has shown that most of the cost of therapy is concentrated in the final months of many terminal patients; in fact, it should be just the opposite, but sadly it's not the case.

Not only the financial burdens are enormous on the dying patient's family, but it's a very emotional time for the family too. A family member is dying, so they feel obligated to do something and sometimes life savings of entire family is sucked up in the last few weeks of the patient's life, as the patient is often in ICU setting, on life support machines.

This needs to change and there are many practitioners who are now embracing the concept of "end of life care" more than ever. After a life ridden with most painful existential experiences, a cancer patient is entitled to at least die in peace.

If intravenous fluids are given at the end of life, then patients have high probability of dying a *wet death,* which is considered much more painful than *dry death,* which occurs when no intravenous fluids are given near end of life. This has been demonstrated in clinical trials, but it's impossibly difficult for a medical professional to just give nothing to a dehydrated, hungry patient and it's even more difficult for the family members, who have to make an informed decision of not administering anything to the dying patient.

Education and communication are the key. Doctors should educate and patients should listen to such honest advice. We should never forget the *primum non nocere.*

CHAPTER 22
SURVIVORSHIP

Only a few other things give me greater joy than to discuss nuances of cancer survivorship with my patients. What it attests to is the effectiveness of cancer treatments and the expertise of myself as a professional.

Many cancers are now curable and many others have acquired the status of a chronic diseases, much like diabetes and hypertension. There are two phases of successful cancer treatment, the treatment itself and the equally important part *surveillance*.

Any discussion of cancer management is incomplete without discussing surveillance. Basically surveillance is done for two purposes: to identify the recurrence or development of another cancer as early as possible and to manage the long term side effects of cancer therapy.

Some chemotherapies given for the treatment of solid tumors may give rise to blood cancers later, with a variable lag time of to two to five years or maybe more. Radiation therapy, especially when given early in adolescence or childhood can give rise to secondary cancers later in life, along with other dysfunctions.

On the other hand, there are cancers which require some form of maintenance therapy, which is continued indefinitely, even after no assessable disease remains. Examples include multiple myeloma, chronic myeloid leukaemia etc. These pose unique challenges in both balancing the ongoing therapy and functionality of the individual.

Patients have the biggest part to play in survivorship. If they stop smoking and embrace healthy lifestyles, like being physically active, avoiding excessive alcohol consumption and others; then studies have consistently shown the decrease in cancer recurrence, reduced rates of development of other cancers and improvement in overall well being.

There are published guidelines for surveillance of every cancer, as well as for healthy lifestyles that the patients should then follow. The combined efforts of oncologists, patients and their families will give the most favourable outcomes.

CHAPTER 23
NOTES ON MYSELF

A quote I often remember is by Churchill, "success is going from failure to failure without losing enthusiasm". I and many of my colleagues face failures everyday and successes too, although most of the times both are relative and seldom absolute.

What I do, I try to do best. But it's hard to put a finger on my best efforts correlating with success. Say, for example, I am treating a patient of extensively metastatic, stage four, relapsed ovarian cancer, then what will actually constitute my success? Trial data are there and newer drugs are very promising, but what is it that I will call my success? Because most of the times, the patient is eventually going to progress and die; it's only a matter of time and I do my best to prolong that time.

In many other specialities success is curing the patient of his ailment, while in medical oncology practice it is very often not the case. We talk about increasing the overall survival or progression free survival in advanced cancer and while it is very rewarding to cure a minority of these advanced patients, many succumb.

In my medical oncology practice, the principles of patient care are the cornerstone. Many times, all I have to do is to listen to the patients and offer my sympathy. The humanitarian aspect of medical oncology practice is more important in my opinion than the academics.

Many oncologists experience *burnout*, which is a term being thrown around loosely these days. Many, in fact, are not burnt out but simply not well adjusted. Burnout is a diagnosis of thorough evaluation, and not every time you feel unhappy and are lost in your search of meaning, should you say that you are burnt out. I believe that oncologists can avoid being burnt out, if they embrace the more spiritual side of human life and see their role as friends of patients rather than being result driven.

We are all after results and I always strive hard to obtain the best possible results; but even then, the most important result for me is the act of practicing wisdom more than knowledge. The actions of listening to the patient, making them feel that they are not alone, being there every time and navigate them through tough choices in face of emotionally demanding situations, are the results I am always after. I can assure my fellow practitioners that burnout will never be there if we get our perspectives right.

Everybody is going to die, cancer patient or otherwise. So if a patient dies, it is not something unexpected or unacceptable, what matters is what you can do to help them live better, before that time comes. I have many relatives of deceased patients of mine who come to me, call me or message me when there is a festivity, invite me to their celebrations; that is the result I'm after. So if the median overall survival of a patient was expected to be three months and he dies in one month, that should not lead to burnout; if you were there and you made it better for the family to bear that time you have done your job and that's a job you and I can always do.

CHAPTER 24

DEMYSTIFICATION

P ractice is so much different than theory. When as a medical student I read textbooks and went through guidelines, it all seemed so complex. And when I became consultant it became even more so. Oncology as a medical speciality is difficult in it's every aspect, and when you add myths and reservation of people to the equation, it becomes very difficult to deal with. There is such a narrow window of opportunity during which cancers can be cured, that every barrier counts. Delay of every week in attaining proper diagnosis and starting treatment is exponentially detrimental.

The large part of my job as a consultant medical oncologist is not to educate my patients about the subtle differences in cancer types, role of genetic testing and their impact or the adverse effect profiles of equally efficacious therapies; but is to dispel, or at least trying to dispel, the entirely unfounded and ever so harmful myths they have. Myths are so widespread, about every aspect of cancer, like *"biopsy will spread my cancer"*, *"chemotherapy causes cancer"*, *"radiation will melt my body"* or *"extensive surgery is worse than death"*. And when I ask my patients about the foundation of their beliefs, they often give answers in anecdotes.

Maybe they had a friend or relative, who took some cancer treatment and didn't get better, maybe they have heard about someone who suffered from too many side effects of chemo or radiation, someone may have died in surgery; these are genuine reasons to be afraid. I always keep reminding myself, because it's so easy to get sidetracked, that the patient or their relatives are not asking these questions for fun, no matter how bizarre these questions may sound to my scientific mind. They ask these questions because they want help, reassurance and proper guidance.

Some of these misconceptions are a result of conditioning in past by personal experiences or by someone else's, some are due to ignorance and others are purposefully spread by nonprofessionals. People have such a hard time coming to terms with their diagnosis that to expect them to let go of their conformations by themselves or even with expert counselling, is too much to ask from them. I always practice patience and empathy.

As a famous neurologist once said that it may be an everyday procedure to perform the neurological examination for the doctor, but it's often the first time for the patient. And the biases in thinking come to play, even for the most experienced doctor. Another aspect that affects counselling and its impact on patient's preconceptions, is the sheer amount of progress that has been made in the field of oncology, and the gaps the small counselling session tries to fill, are almost impossible to bridge. Most of the people use smartphones and they are not experts in electronics and electromagnetism, but they have a working practical knowledge. On the other hand, there is seldom anyone so practically informed of cancer therapeutics.

The list of myths and misinformed notions is endless and it is beyond the scope of this book to discuss each one individually. A simple answer is thus needed, and it is: *it depends*. The real problem lies not in the questions but the answers. There is no definitive answer to any myth, as it's not possible to draw a negative conclusion with certainty most of the time. If I say naturopathy can't cure stage four lung cancer, how am I going to prove it?

So, it's better to ask questions to your doctor or any other health professional or any other practitioner for that matter, and ask for evidence to back the claims they are making. Honesty is the best policy and the most important one too. If your doctor answers *"we don't know"* or *"a large scale study has failed to show"* or *"there is not enough evidence"*, then that's the truth and it's verifiable too. Grandiose claims are easy to make, it's easy to fall for such claims too. But an indeterminate answer given scientifically, is better than an outright lie.

My take on demystifying cancer is providing the best available knowledge to a particular question, with concrete data to back what I am saying. Rest is upto the patient. Scientific knowledge by its nature is ever evolving and surely getting better with time. It's ok to not know an answer. What's more important is to rely on answers that we do have for certain questions and capitalize on those.

One example is the indisputable benefit of HER2 directed therapies in a subset of metastatic breast cancer patients, recent trials have shown median overall survival of 56 months in these patients using certain drug combinations compared to 40 months with other combinations and much less with other, more *conventional* methods. These are facts, available for everyone to read and improve upon. What about triple negative breast cancers then? We don't have enough data for making recommendations, that are universally applicable for such stage four patients, but trials are showing results and soon there will be answers. This kind of discussion is better and progressive than just saying *"drink this potion and you will live for a hundred years"*.

We, as a society, should focus more on the facts than fiction and more on concrete data than anecdotes. If someone tells you that one of their relatives has gotten rid of leukemia by going on a certain diet and supplement concoction, then more power to them. But ask for data and governmental policies. I know many people, in fact, I deal with such people everyday, who demonize modern medicine and question the authenticity of governmental regulatory bodies. My question is, how do you then trust some random person who makes a claim without any scientific testing and published data, thereby potentially endangering people's lives? What are the parameters by which you judge the authenticity of such *"miraculous remedies"*?

CHAPTER 25
RESOURCE POOR SETTINGS

My colleagues and I often have this discussion, it's true to some extent that cancer is a disease of the rich. What we mean by that is, the kind of money needed to properly diagnose and treat cancer patients is enormous. Even internationally accepted guidelines, like NCCN, publish separate guidelines for resource poor settings.

In my country, it is a common story: a patient walks into the clinic, I tell him about the investigations, the charges and although I work in a charitable hospital, where rates of procedures and medicines are nominal, even then patients refuse any form of treatment directed to their cancer and insist on just symptomatic medicines. Many government and semi-government hospitals are in place and so are many patient assistance programs, but they are far from enough.

One of my seniors always said *"it's easy to get the first remission or to decrease the size of any cancerous lump, but it is painstakingly difficult to actually cure the cancer"*. Many types of cancer therapies are there which are not the standard of care, but they can get the job done for a while. Famously in medical oncology practice, if a patient of lymphoma is given nothing but steroids the lumps that they have got may sometimes nearly disappear. Similarly in acute lymphoblastic leukaemia, following a less intense protocol along with steroids, can send the patient into remission, but only for a few weeks to months. These things are practiced in resource poor settings and they do more harm than good.

That's a sad reality that due to lack of resources many very much curable cancer patients are dying every day. Then there are the patented drugs and the sky high prices. I am not an expert of medical policy making but I am an expert of oncology. When I started my MBBS, I never thought much about the *big pharma,* but with the passage of years, I have come to an understanding that they are a necessary evil.

So much research is going on in medical oncology and almost everything is driven by pharma companies. This is leading to breakthroughs at a prolific rate, which is very good. But the question glaring before me is what am I to say to the man sitting in front of me, the mother of whom has stage four lung cancer and who is earning just enough to buy food for his family day after day? How can he afford latest tyrosine kinase inhibitors or immunotherapy molecules?

It's easy to say that policy should be made but the more I dwell on this subject the more perplexed I get. Many of the drugs that are now the talk of the day, are out of even my reach if I have to buy them for my own use. It breaks my heart and I wish there was a way to deal with it.

CHAPTER 26

PAIN IS REAL

To conclude, I should now leave oncology behind and talk about the challenges that are sometimes insurmountable. It is a glorious feat to prevent cancer, very satisfying when we are able to detect cancer at earliest stages and completely cure the patient, and the almost unbelievable survival benefits of modern medicines are a blessing, but that's not the point. What about those who suffer and suffer a lot? You know, there are days when I just want to leave my profession and there are days when I am so ecstatic that I want to be an oncologist more than anything, and I want my child to also be an oncologist.

The reality is that majority of patients, especially in developing countries, have so many barriers to healthcare that the situation is hopeless from the day they first consult and sometimes they don't consult at all. Most of the times, I know that all that I am going to do will just be exercises in futility. On the other hand, even if the best of the best medical care is provided, still many patients either don't get cured or relapse. I am not a hardcore researcher, I am a practicing medical oncologist, but people don't go to research labs. They come to doctors for getting treatment and end their suffering.

I always consider it my first and foremost duty to treat the *patient* and not just the *disease.* So many doctors, for whatever reasons, get so much trapped in treating the disease that the patient is completely forgotten. Every cycle of chemo is analysed like a mathematical problem, with grading of adverse effects being done, the responses being evaluated and all that. While it's true that doctors are pressed for time, I have seen more patient satisfaction when I remember their names without looking at the files, taking mental notes of a few important aspects of their personal lives and keeping track of those and most importantly, trying to give them this sense of me being there as a friend and guardian whenever they need me.

In today's world, it's hard to practice medicine, as lawsuits are plenty and every wrong outcome is considered to be the doctor's fault, but I let go of all this negativity. I know that it's always easy to practice humanity, in fact, it is a must.

www.ingramcontent.com/pod-product-compliance
Lightning Source LLC
Chambersburg PA
CBHW021236280526
45784CB00005B/2120